I0423958

# Vaccine Free Healthy in a Viral Epidemic

## How to Prevent Virus Infections Vaccine-Free with Three Effective Antiviral Strategies

Traudl Woehlke

All rights reserved. No part of this book may be
reproduced or used in any way or form or by any
means whether electronic or mechanical without the
prior written consent of the publisher.
© 2016 Sunrise-Verlag

1st edition 2016
Printed in USA

1

Dear Reader,

Congratulations and thanks for getting my book. You are one of the increasing number of people who are looking for safe and effective natural solutions for health and well-being. People like you make this world a better place.

Let's spread the news of the power of natural cures and prevention. There is no need for panic and fear when you are informed!

Please leave a review on Amazon to help others discover how they can help themselves in a safe way.
Thanks.

Traudl Woehlke
Contact: Rawfoodforyou3@gmail.com

*Books by Traudl Wöhlke*

Raw Food for Babies                     Raw Food in
for Happier, Healthier Infants          Pregnancy

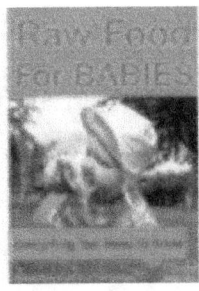 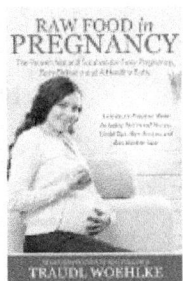

# About

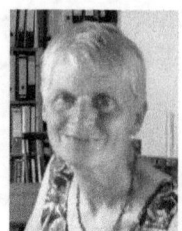 Traudl Woehlke is a licensed German healing practitioner specializing in homeopathy, whole and raw food nutrition and energy psychology. It has been her mission to empower her readers to take control of their health by providing relevant information anybody can apply.

Traudl lives in Southern Germany. She is mother to two adult daughters, "grandmother" to a dozen horses and foster mother to 6 stray cats. She loves to be outdoors, foraging all edibles to be found in nature.

She has lived on whole and raw foods with her family for more than 30 years, and taught whole and raw food nutrition for decades to adults and kids. After she experienced the benefits of homeopathy in her kids, her animals and herself, she studied and trained in homeopathy and qualified for a formal healing license.

She is available for health and nutritional consultations via email and Skype.

Contact: Rawfoodforyou3@gmail.com

# Table of Contents

# Introduction

DID YOU KNOW?

The CDC reported in 2014 that the flu vaccines were ineffective because they did not address the current virus strain. It takes six months to develop a vaccine. That's why producing the right type of vaccines to address the ever mutating viruses is like gambling. You just don't know what specific influenza virus will be in season at the time of vaccine production.

Now what do you do to protect yourself against viral infections? Avoid crowds? Wear facial protective masks? Boost your immunity? Take vitamin supplements?

In fact, there are scientifically proven successful ways of preventing viral infections naturally vaccine-free. This booklet outlines in detail the three most effective options. You will find out what you can do to stay healthy in any epidemic.

The content of this booklet is based on the research and clinical experience of Dr. B. Sandler's MD and Dr. M. O. Bruker MD. You too can benefit from Dr Sandler's research and experience. All you need to know is outlined in "Vaccine Free Healthy in a Viral Epidemic".
The booklet is an abridged version of Dr B Sandler's findings updated with the more recent knowledge and

60 years' clinical experience of the German doctor M O Bruker MD.

In addition, it also reveals the little known but proven power of homeopathy in preventing and treating even severe virus epidemics.

Also, you'll find detailed actionable advice and guidelines on how simple lifestyle changes can make all the difference in your health.

To your health!

# 1 – Viruses and Viral Infections

Viruses! Just mentioning the word gives you the shivers!

Human viruses often are very contagious and new strands appear monthly. So far about 2000 varieties are known. This can be pretty scary as some severe diseases are related to viral infections such as hepatitis, polio, AIDS, and influenza (flu). Many childhood diseases are caused by viruses such as the measles, chickenpox, German measles, and mumps. Viral infections do not respond to antibiotic treatment. Vaccines were developed to prevent viral illnesses.

## Viral Infections And Their Effects

Viruses are capable of being transferred by air, or by being swallowed or inhaled (influenza), by sexual contact (AIDS) or via the transfer of body fluids such as blood (hepatitis), even by insects (e. g. West Nile virus). More commonly, viruses are transmitted from mucous and saliva through coughing, sneezing, biting and spitting. So there seems to be no way of avoiding exposure to viruses.

Viruses usually infect one particular type of cell. For example, cold viruses infect only cells of the upper respiratory tract. Additionally, most viruses infect only a few species of plants or animals. Some infect only people, others infect animals and are transferred to humans such as rabies.

## Most Common Types of Viral Infections

The most common viral infections are those of the nose, throat, and the upper airway. These infections include sore throat, sinusitis, and the common cold. Influenza is a viral respiratory infection. Some viruses, such as rabies, West Nile virus, and several different encephalitis viruses, infect the nervous system. Viral infections also develop in the skin, sometimes resulting in warts, shingles or rashes.

Other common viral infections are caused by herpes viruses. Eight different herpes viruses infect people. Three of them—herpes simplex virus type 1 and type 2, and varicella-zoster virus—cause infections that produce blisters on the skin or mucus membranes. Another herpes virus, Epstein-Barr virus, causes infectious mononucleosis.

## Understanding Viruses

Viruses are tiny infectious organisms which invade a living cell to reproduce resulting in infection. In this case, it attaches to a cell, enters it, and releases its genetic material (DNA or RNA) inside the cell. The virus' DNA or RNA contains the information needed to reproduce the virus. The virus' genetic material takes control of the host cell and forces it to replicate the virus. Now, you are sick. Luckily we are equipped with our immune system which fights viral attacks and is capable of destroying the virus.

## Immune Responses to Viral Attack

Most viruses enter the body through your mouth and nose. Some enter through a break in the skin such as a bite. Inside the body, they may encounter phagocytic white blood cells. The role of this type of blood cell is to engulf and digest the viruses.

If viruses avoid capture, they may cause development of a special group of proteins. These proteins called antibodies are very specific. They attack the invading virus and attach to it. The virus is destroyed by the antibody directly or held until it can be surrounded by white blood cells.

If a virus does invade a cell, it sets off a chemical alarm. Another group of proteins called interferons are produced when a cell is invaded. Interferons are released from infected cells and bind to the membranes of neighboring cells. These neighboring cells are now protected from invading viruses.

Interferons are produced when any virus invades a cell. The interferon produced by one species will not work in another.

## Viruses Outsmart the Immune System

With every replication, the virus changes its genetic make-up. At least one of its genes mutates and new virus strands appears with new qualities. This is how the virus outsmarts the immune system. Our body needs to create new resistance to detect and fight the virus. And for that reason, vaccines must constantly be adjusted to address these new strands.

## Effects on Infected Cells

When some viruses keep the infected cell from performing its normal function, we become ill, and the infected cell dies. When an infected cell dies, it releases new viruses which go on to infect other cells.

Not all viruses kill the cells they infect, but instead alter the cell's functions. Sometimes the infected cell loses control over normal cell division. Evidence now points to certain viral groups as high risk factors in some cancerous conditions. However, other genetic and environmental factors are necessary before a virus can cause cancer.

All herpes viruses cause lifelong infection because the virus remains within its host cell in a dormant state (latent infection). Typically, the

11

virus reactivates and produces further episodes of disease when your immune system is in a weakened condition. Reactivation may occur rapidly or many years after the initial infection.

## Good Virus Infections

Not all virus infections are bad. Certain virus infections are capable of beating cancer. Parvovirus HL1 is one. This virus attaches to tumor cells and destroys only those leaving the healthy cells uninflected.

Other useful viruses control the algae growth in the sea or fight bacteria in commercially bred lobster replacing antibiotics.

# Antiviral Drugs

Your immune system fights a viral infection naturally. However, antibiotics have no effect on a virus. In most cases, a virus simply has to run its course. There are certain instances when antiviral drugs are prescribed by a doctor. Most of these drugs function not by killing the virus directly, but rather by interfering with its ability to reproduce itself.

Antiviral drugs are rather limited in scope, in part because viral infections come in many different forms and are known for their frequent mutations. As mentioned before, a virus is highly specialized just like a lock and a key. This makes it hard to keep up with the changes. The science is very complex and costly. Therefore, the best approach is to prevent viral infections.

It all comes down to preventing a viral infection. Standard medicine pushes vaccines for prevention. Other options are strengthening the immune system naturally. In the following sections of this report you will find detailed actionable advice on how to prevent any virus infection even in times of epidemics.

# 2 - Health Risks of Vaccines and Antiviral Medication

## Vaccines

In the US, the government and conventional medical agencies vigorously promote vaccinations with the promise of disease prevention. People who question the veracity of vaccines pose these questions:

- Why is a budget of 2 billion dollars needed to financially compensate vaccine-injured children?
- Why are pediatricians exempted by law from legal liability for any vaccine damage inflicted upon a child?
- Why is there a lack of information on safe disease prevention?

Like prescription drugs, vaccines are pharmaceutical products carrying risks: the risk the product doesn't work and the risk the product causes harm. One would expect vaccines recommended and enforced upon a population are risk-free. Unfortunately, neither vaccines nor antiviral medication are completely safe to use. So it's up to those who are potential recipients of a vaccine to understand the complications.

## Do Vaccines Work?

Do vaccines work? Not always and not in the way you would expect.

During a 1976 polio epidemic in Israel, 50% of the infected children had been vaccinated 3 to 4 times. Another disturbing condition is that people who were vaccinated have infected others without being sick themselves. Another example of an ineffective vaccine is occurred in Hungary. In 1981, 60% of those that had contracted the measles had been fully vaccinated. In 1989, in the US an entire school population of vaccinated children, 4,200 students, succumbed to measles.

The ineffectiveness of vaccines continues to be a strong argument against them. Certain types of vaccines had to be withdrawn from use either because of their adverse side effects or because they just didn't work. In 1992, in the UK a combo-vaccine covering measles, mumps, and German measles was withdrawn from the market.

Unfortunately, it took four years before recognizing the adverse side effects.

## Harmful Effects of Vaccines

### Individual Reaction to Vaccines

Every individual reacts different to vaccination. Some individuals will show no side effects. However, others may be adversely affected even suffering from incurable health damage for a lifetime. There is no way of predicting how the individual will react to vaccines. According to the German physician Dr. Buchwald the risk of contracting health damage by vaccines is higher than catching the viral disease you are trying to prevent by vaccines.

When a viral infection is overcome naturally without interference of vaccines, you are rewarded with lifelong immunity. You also aren't subjected to the inherent risks of using a vaccine. This is why holistic doctors consider childhood diseases a good thing for children as overcoming them naturally strengthens a child's immune system. Without a vaccine, a child can contract a childhood disease only once in a lifetime because its immune system has created antibodies that will fight any future viral attacks.

## Examples Of Vaccine Reactions And Vaccine Damage

Below are examples of some very detrimental health conditions which occurred after a vaccination.

Adverse reactions to a vaccine may show right after the inoculation or a week or longer later. They range from mild to severe to the point of disabling an individual mentally and/or physically for a lifetime.

With children, short-term vaccine reactions may present immediately or within a week to include: crying, irritability, high pitched screaming, excessive sleeping, ear infections, eczema, deafness, encephalitis (brain inflammation), Shaken Baby Syndrome, sudden infant death. Adverse long-term vaccine reactions in children are known to cause Autism, Aspergers, ADHD/ADD, as well as neurological complications such as seizures, multiple sclerosis, Guillain Barre Syndrom (disturbed immune system and paralysis), and immunological reactions.

Adults are not without health risks with vaccinations. Consider these possible reactions to flu shots: mild short-term reactions include soreness, redness, and swelling at the injection site, fainting, headache, nausea, muscle ache, vomiting, fever. Possible serious side effects of flu vaccination include difficulty in breathing, hoarseness, swelling around the eyes or lips, hives, paleness, weakness, racing heart, dizziness, behavior changes, and/or high fever.

## Vaccine Ingredients

The toxic and allergenic ingredients used during vaccine production can pose health risks. Vaccines may be contaminated with or may be composed of viruses, fetal tissue, mycoplasma, cancer cells, DNA/RNA, BSE, genetic engineering, Mercury/ Thimerosal, adjuvants such as Aluminum and Squalene, and other substances. (For a more detailed explanation visit http://www.whale.to/vaccine/vaccinemyth.pdf)

To calculate your personal toxin load that you have picked up by your vaccinations, go to the vaccine calculator at 4) http://www.vaccine-tlc.org/vic.

Medical and governmental agencies have denied risks associated with vaccines. At the same time, the FDA, CDC and vaccine makers admit that often the number of human subjects used in pre-licensing studies are too small to detect rarer adverse events, making post-marketing surveillance of new vaccines a de facto scientific experiment.
There is no research in the long-term effects of vaccines.

One study was done in Italy In 1996. It discovered biochemical markers of vaccine damage. There is no other research in this field known. You can access the study here:

5) http://www.whale.to/v/coulter3.html

## Vaccine Injury Compensation

The National Vaccine Information Center worked with the U.S. Congress on the National Childhood Vaccine Injury Act of 1986. This act acknowledged vaccine injuries and deaths are real and those injured by vaccines should be financially compensated.

As a result of the Vaccine Injury Act of 1986, over $2 billion compensation has been awarded to children and adults injured by vaccines. The law preserved the right for vaccine injured persons to bring a lawsuit in the court system if federal compensation is denied or is not sufficient. By 2010, the U.S. Court of Claims had awarded nearly $2 billion dollars to vaccine victims for their catastrophic vaccine injuries, although two out of three applicants have been denied compensation.

(Refer to 6) http://www.nvic.org/injury-compensation.aspx)

## Antiviral Medication

Antiviral medication presents risks, too. Antiviral drugs can be toxic to human cells. Viruses can develop resistance to antiviral drugs. Known side effects include nausea, vomiting, diarrhea, headache, rashes, kidney damage, confusion, loss of appetite, nervousness, unsteadiness, sleeplessness, low white blood cell count, electrolyte disturbances, seizures, anemia, flu-like symptoms, depression, dizziness, breakdown of red blood cells causing anemia, stinging of the eyes, swelling of the eyelids, sensitivity to light, as well as irritation of the airways

# 3 – Early Discoveries of Prevention

## Polio in Asheville - The Discoveries of Dr. Benjamin Sandler, M.D.

Dr. Sandler was an American polio researcher. He discovered in the 1940's that polio (a virus) was associated with an individual's blood sugar level fall below its physiological level. Dr. Sandler put this discovery to use, and spread his knowledge in a public campaign in Ashville, N. C. during a polio epidemic.

Dr. Sandler discovered that blood sugar below the norm was a pre-requisite to viral infection. Accorddingly, to stay healthy in a viral epidemic, Sandler taught to avoid participation in anything which caused blood sugar levels to drop.

He observed that strenuous physical activities such as participating in athletic contests and swimming in cold water lower blood sugar below the norm.

The same holds true for eating **refined / simple** carbohydrates such as sugar, ice-cream, soft-drinks, canned fruit, cookies, cakes, candy, along with standard bread, noodles, white rice, white flour and any food products containing refined sugar and flour.

Therefore Dr. Sandler recommended a diet without simple carbohydrates (mainly refined sugar and flour) and to refrain from strenuous physical activities.

The media supported Sandler's recommendations and spread the word throughout the community. People followed Dr. Sandler's advice and avoided a large scale spread of polio.

Ashville was spared from the polio epidemic as long as the media supported Dr. Sandler's recommendations. People followed the advice and saved the newspaper clips covering details and shared it with friends in other areas.

However, the next epidemic could not be prevented on a large scale because the media no longer informed about Dr. Sandler's recommendations due to the influence of the ice-cream industry.

**60 Years of Dr. M. O. Bruker's Clinical Practice**

Dr. M. O. Bruker M. D. was a German physician and homeopath specializing in internal medicine. He combined the knowledge of Dr. Sandler with the findings of other researchers spanning sixty years of clinical practice with more than 40,000 patients. Dr. Bruker promoted a diet of whole and raw foods including whole grains (complex carbohydrates) in the hospitals he managed. He found that whole grains balance blood sugar and prevent spikes with their extreme ups and downs.

# 4 - Simple Strategies to Prevent Viral Infections

This section is all about risk free, safe ways for preventing the flu and other viral infections. These methods are proven to work. They come without side effects and they improve your immunity, as well as your overall health. They are inexpensive. Nevertheless, there is no way of guaranteeing good health. However, the likelihood of avoiding viral infections is positive when you follow the practical advice outlined in this chapter.

Keeping your blood sugar balanced within its normal range is the key of prevention. So what causes low blood sugar in humans? Most common weaknesses are due to dietary errors.

Additionally, extreme physical exertion combined with eating sweets, stress and emotional unrest causes blood sugar to plummet.

## The Importance of Diet

## Foods to Eat, Foods to Avoid

As mentioned before, diet is the single most health factor. Even if you still are on the standard American diet, if you want to stay healthy in an epidemic,

- then avoid junk food, refined sugar and flour, starches, juices, canned fruits, cooked fruits, jam, ice cream, syrups, nectars, anything that is not naturally sweet but has sweeteners added.
- Adopt eating "clean" also known as "whole food" menus. This strengthens your immunity and overall health and prevents fluctuations of blood sugar. A clean diet includes fresh vegetables, some fresh fruits, whole grains, and foods made of whole grains such as whole grain bread, whole grain noodles, brown rice, nuts, seeds, oil fruits, butter, fresh whipped and sour cream, and cold pressed unrefined vegetable oils.
- Use fresh and whole ingredients every meal. A minimum of one third of your food intake needs to be raw vegetables.

Any (refined) sugar you consume in food and beverages, will rapidly lower blood sugar. This is a physiological reaction. On whole grains, there are no extreme drops, and you won't get into a stage that makes you prone for viral infections nor will you experience this urge for sweets which is common when you are on the standard American diet.

When your blood sugar is low, you tend to search for sweets to make you feel better. If you follow your craving, the cycle of peaks and subsequent drops of blood sugar is going on and on – like an addiction. Have you ever noticed about an hour after eating refined sugar and flour/starches, you become sleepy. This is a sure sign your blood sugar has dropped. *The level remains low* for one to two hours while the meal is digested. *This is the timeframe when you are prone to viral infections.*

## Physical Exertion in Moderation During Epidemics

Physical exertion also causes moderate to severe fall of blood sugar. The recommendations below are to help prevent drops in blood sugar levels. In order to keep your body strong during a flu or other type of epidemic, *avoid intense physical activity.* Extreme physical exertion as found in athletic contests, drills and the like should be avoided during epidemics. Short periods of exercise are fine.

Football players, marathon runners, tennis players, boxers, swimmers... pro or amateur athletes are more at risk because they usually workout with extreme physical exertion. They usually compete with others which adds another risk. Very fit and healthy individuals have been reported to catch a virus infection within 24 hours after physical exertion.

## Avoid swimming in cold water.
Your blood sugar and the glycogen levels are depleted while the body adapts to the cold water trying to return the body temperature to a normal state. Glycogen is blood sugar stored in the liver to make blood sugar available to the cells at all times.

## Avoid Eating Ice--Cream when you are out at the beach or pool swimming.
The combination of cooling your body when swimming and eating the sugar loaded ice-cream depletes your blood sugar and the glycogen levels the most, putting you at very high risk of viral infection.

## Sufficient Rest and Keep Warm
Make sure to get adequate rest and restorative sleep Keep warm, make sure your feet are warm. Why? Warm feet are well supplied with blood, and the blood flow of your feet correlates with the blood flow of your head. This means when there is good blood flow in your feet (your feet are warm), it will be the same in in the mucus tissue

of your head. Why does this matter? A good blood flow greatly improves the functtion of your immune system. It carries fresh blood enriched with oxygen and nutrients to the tissue and removes toxins and waste. This is important as mouth and nose are the area of first contact with many viruses. You want to make sure the virus gets defeated as fast as possible.

One of the easiest ways to get warm feet is brisk walking, or even a few minutes of rope jumping, if you cannot make it outdoors. Another very effective way is a rising foot bath where you alternate very warm and very cold water ending with cold water.

When in bed, wet socks are a great way to get your feet warm, and to improve your circulation.

## Spices To Improve Immunity

### Cayenne Peppers

If you are aware of your body, you will most likely notice when you are about to catch a cold. You feel tired, and unwell, before you are actually ill. If you catch this early phase, cayenne peppers may take care of the beginning cold for good. Just eat 3 to 5 (or more to your liking) peppers immediately, and continue eating a few more later in the day and the next one to two days, and you may be all set without contracting the cold.

Notice: This only works at the very onset of a cold.

You need not take the hottest pepper for the desired effect. Mild peppers, and even pickled and marinated kinds can work.

To be prepared and for fast action, you may want to keep some cayenne peppers in your pantry.

Cayenne, also known as capsicin, opens the bronchial passages, and increases blood flow and is an anti-inflammatory. Its ingredients help your body produce white blood cells, build healthy mucus membrane tissue that defends against viruses and bacteria. Spicy cayenne peppers raise your body's temperature to make you sweat, increasing the activity of your immune system.

## Garlic & Co.

Fresh raw garlic, fresh cut raw onion, fresh raw horseradish root, and fresh ginger are the spices you should be using daily during an epidemic. They all stimulate your immune system as research has shown. However, they cannot make up the health risks of the standard American diet.

## Avoid Emotional Distress: Tapping for Fast Relief

Stress and worries increase your susceptibility to viral infections. It is not always possible to do away with it. An easy way for emotional balance and immediate relief is tapping. Tapping has been described as emotional acupuncture without needles. There are dozens of tapping video tutorials on YouTube. The practice is easy to learn and a proven therapy for removing all types of physical and emotional distress.

9) Tapping http://www.eftdownunder.com/videos/

In addition, observe common sense rules such as

- Avoid events where you participate as a player or fan.
- Reduce your contact with others who may be carrying the virus.
- Avoid crowds.

# 5 – Homeopathic Prevention and Treatment of Viral Infections

Homeopathy isn't home remedies, herbs, or naturopathy, or a harmless drug. Instead it is a powerful scientific method of treatment based on the universal law of similar meaning like cures like. It is radically different from any other system of medicine, and has been proven effective, and gentle since 1796 on every continent. Homeopathy is used all over the world to treat humans, animals and plants with impressive results in acute and even severe chronic conditions, and in epidemics.

There is a lot of recent research that confirms the homeopathic approach.
Professor Luc Montagnier, French virologist and Nobel laureate says: *"What I can say now is that high dilutions are right. High dilutions of something are not nothing. They are water structures that mimic the original molecules. It's not pseudo-science. It's not quackery. These are real phenomena which deserve further studies."*

Homeopathy is a safe alternative for vaccines and antiviral drugs. It has a long recorded history of successful treatment and prevention of viral infections and epidemics in many countries all over the world. Homeopathy has become one of the three pillars of the official Indian medical system.

In India, homeopaths successfully prevented the outbreak of a severe measles epidemic by administering the matching homeopathic remedy to everyone in the risk area.

In 1996, Cuba prevented the outbreak of a much feared seasonal epidemic in a similar way. In 2006, Brazil implemented homeopathy in the public health service because of its success in preventing and treating Dengue epidemics. In the US, until 1920, homeopathy was very common, and homeopathic doctors were hugely successful curing and preventing epidemics without side effects. Statistics show that their treatment was superior to conventional treatment.

Unlike any other therapeutic system, homeopathy stimulates a person's inherent healing force which gently restores health surprisingly fast. Homeopathic prescription considers the individual particularities of a patient, and its remedies are low-cost.

It is possible for lay people to learn to use homeopathy on their own. Throughout the history of homeopathy, it's been lay people who ensured the survival of homeopathy when it was under attack of established medicine.

In our day and age, it is especially valuable for those without health insurance. It is a powerful system of natural medicine at low cost that works for humans, animals and plants alike.

## Homeopathy for Flu Prevention

When the flu is rampant in your neighborhood, consider using a homeopathic prophylactic against it. One of the best is Influenzinum 30 C. You can begin this approximately one month before flu season starts by giving four doses four times in one day Repeat this every week for one month. Stop when the threat is over.

This prophylactic is usually highly effective, but if you develop a fever or scratchy throat, take Oscillococcium every four hours for two to three days. This remedy is one of the most popular over-the-counter flu remedies sold in Europe and has a reputation for stopping an illness in its tracks or considerably shortening its duration. This remedy is particularly effective for a cold or flu that comes on in cold, wet weather.

Influenzinum is made from the vaccine from the seasonal vaccine of this year or from previous years. Influenzinum is more effective than the vaccine as shown in a study with 30 people.

In India, many epidemics have been prevented and treated in this way such as measles and cholera. Recently, Cuba, Brazil and other countries also have been widely successful in preventing serious seasonal epidemics of leptospirosis, hepatitis, dengue fever, malaria by giving everyone at risk highly diluted pathogens just like homeopathic remedies are produced, the efficacy of this procedure was outstanding. No side-effects have ever been reported.

Not only are the results outstanding, also the costs to produce those medicines are extremely low, just 3% of the costs of producing vaccines. And the homeopathic-style remedies can be produced within two weeks whereas it takes six months to come up with a relevant vaccine.

## How to Treat the Flu Using Homeopathy

There are three types of flu. One mainly affects the upper airways and the head, including nose and throat, another type affects digestion and you feel sick to the stomach, and the third type comes with bone and limbs pain. Below you'll find the treatment protocols for all three influenza types as prescribed by the famous Indian homeopaths Drs. Banerji in Kolkotta: 17)

The first line remedies right at the very onset of the flu are Rhus troxicodendron 30C and Bryonia 30C. 2 pills of each of these remedies are to be taken every 2 hours. You start out with one, 2 hours later you take the other, another 2 hours later you take the first one etc.

With **high fever** (102°F), add Belladonna 3C diluted in water, 1 teaspoon every hour. Make the dilution by adding 3 pills Belladonna 3C in a glass of water, stir vigorously with a spoon, and take.1 teaspon of it per dose.

Incase the flu comes with **nausea and vomiting**, add Arsencium album 30C diluted in water, and take one teaspone of the dilution every 30 minutes until improvement.

With **painful bones and limbs** follow this protocol:
You need Eupatorium perfoliatum mother tincture and Bryonia 30C, both remedies to be taken

alternating every 3 hours as described above. One dose of the tincture is 5 drops, one dose of Bryonia is 2 pills.

Incase of **acute sneezing und running nose**, take 2 pills of Arsenicum album 6C every 30 minutes until improvement.

To improve your **overall immunity**, take 2 pills of Calcarea carbonica 30C once a day for several months.

## Where to Find Homeopathic Remedies

There are several homeopathic laboratories that produce FDA approved homeopathic remedies. They are available in health food stores and on the internet.

# 6 - Summary

If you rely on the procedures of standard medicine to prevent and treat viral infections, homeopaths believe your health is at risk. Alternatively, there are proven ways to avoid virus infections and improve your immunity with a clean diet. Moderate lifestyle changes in an epidemic will most likely keep you healthy. While improving your diet and adjusting your lifestyle is solely up to you, safe and effective homeopathic treatment by a qualified homeopath is both a natural and effective alternative.

# Keys to Preventing Viral Infections – Vaccine Free

- Adopt a whole food diet, avoid sugars, and processed foods.
- Avoid intense physical activity, crowds, and keep your feet warm.
- Get to bed and sleep
- Avoid emotional distress, tap if needed

# References

1) Virologist Antonio Marchine. Deutsches Krebsforschungszentrum (German cancer research center)

2) Thomas Quak MD: Impfungen und Impffolgen
http://www.doktor-quak.de/pdf/tq_impfungen.pdf

3) Ingredients of Vaccines
http://www.whale.to/vaccine/vaccinemyth.pdf

4) Vaccine Calculator http://www.vaccine-tlc.org/vic

5) Italian Study on Vaccine Damage
http://www.whale.to/v/coulter3.html

6) Vaccine Injury Compensation
http://www.nvic.org/injury-compensation.aspx

7) Benjamin Sandler MD: Diet Prevents Polio

8) M. O. Bruker MD
http://www.amazon.de/Vollwertern%C3%A4hrung-sch%C3%BCtzt-vor-Viruserkrankungen-Kinderl%C3%A4hmung/dp/3891890176/ref=sr_1_27?s=books&ie=UTF8&qid=1409044507&sr=1-27&keywords=M.+O.+Bruker

9) Tapping http://www.eftdownunder.com/videos/

10) http://www.kostas-
homeopathy.com/homeopathy-explained-
2/homeopathy-in-epidemics/

11) http://hpathy.com/homeopathy-
papers/homoeopathic-immunisation-against-
leptospirosis-in-cuba/

12) http://hpathy.com/homeopathy-
papers/homoeoprophylaxis-historical-snapshot/

13)http://www.ncbi.nlm.nih.gov/pubmed?term=%E2
%80%A2Large-scale%20application%20of%20highly-
diluted%20bacteria%20for%20Leptospirosis%20epide
mic%20control[all]&cmd=correctspelling

14) http://www.homeopathycenter.org/treatment-
epidemics-homeopathy-history

15) Bracho G, Varela E, Fernández R, et al. Large-scale
application of highly-diluted bacteria for Leptospirosis
epidemic control. Homeopathy. 2010; 99: 156-

16) André Saine: Statistics in Homeopathy

17) Prasanta Banerji, Pratip Banerji: The Banerji
Protocols.2013, 89

## Publisher's Note

This publication is intended to provide helpful and informative material. It is not intended to diagnose, treat, cure or prevent any health problem or condition, nor is it intended to replace the advice of a physician. No action should be taken solely on the contents of this book. Always consult your physician or qualified health-care professional on any matters regarding your health and before adopting any suggestions in this book or drawing inferences from it.

The author and publisher specifically disclaim all responsibility for any liability, loss or risk, personal or otherwise, which is incurred as a consequence, directly or indirectly, from the use or application of any contents of this book.

Dear Reader,

Thank you for reading this book. I take all efforts to bring well-researched and useful content to you.

Please let me know if this book has been of value to you. Any of your suggestions and ideas are very much appreciated.

You may contact me for any questions that have not been answered in this book at rawfoodpublishing@gmail.com .

Please leave your review on Amazon.

Thanks.

Traudl Woehlke

www.ingramcontent.com/pod-product-compliance
Lightning Source LLC
Chambersburg PA
CBHW061932280526
45787CB00004B/1573